Petriv

"Learned more than I expected with 'Testicular Talks'. A gem!" - Zoe Fitzpatrick

"'Guardians of Genetics' is brilliantly written and well-researched." - Tasha Williams

"The 'Dual Dilemma' addresses modern issues with care and nuance. Highly recommend!" - Elijah Kim

NUTS & BOLTS

The Male Reproductive System Uncovered

Disclaimer:

The information provided in "Nuts and Bolts: The Male Reproductive System Uncovered" is intended for general knowledge purposes only. It is not a substitute for professional medical advice or treatment. Readers are encouraged to consult with qualified health care professionals regarding any health or medical concerns.

978-1-4467-6277-6
Imprint: Lulu.com

To all the inquisitive minds that strive for understanding, and to the educators and mentors who enlighten paths and inspire journeys.

FOREWORD

When Robert Petriv approached me to pen the foreword for "Nuts and Bolts: The Male Reproductive System Uncovered," I was both honored and curious. My familiarity with Robert's scholarship and depth of knowledge had always left me in awe. Yet, this work promised to delve into territories not just of science and anatomy, but of culture, identity, and human experience.

From the dawn of civilization, the human reproductive system has been shrouded in a mixture of reverence, mystery, and taboo. It has been depicted in art, sung about in songs, and explored in medical literature. But Robert's exploration is distinct. It's not merely a physiological journey into the mechanics of the male reproductive system. It's a sociocultural odyssey, an intimate dance with identity, and a profound reflection on legacy and lineage.

As you leaf through these pages, you'll be taken on a journey that transcends time and space. From the ancient understanding of male virility to the cutting-edge research of today, from the quiet villages where manhood ceremonies still prevail to the bustling cities where modern pressures redefine masculinity, this book bridges worlds.

But what stands out most prominently is the vulnerability and authenticity with which Robert approaches the subject. This is not just a textbook; it's a heartfelt exploration, a compassionate conversation, a tribute to the myriad experiences that define the male reproductive journey.

I've had the privilege of knowing Robert as a colleague and friend. His commitment to deep, holistic understanding, his passion for dispelling myths, and his profound respect for every individual's unique journey shine brilliantly through this work.

In "Nuts and Bolts," Robert has crafted a masterpiece that is both timely and timeless. Whether you approach this work with curiosity, seeking knowledge, or with a personal quest for understanding, you'll emerge enriched, enlightened, and, perhaps, with a renewed sense of wonder about the intricate dance of life.

To Robert, I offer my heartfelt congratulations on this monumental work. To you, the reader, I offer a promise: you're about to embark on a journey that will touch not just your mind, but your heart and soul.

With deepest respect,

Eric Bis

The male reproductive system is an intricate ensemble of organs, glands, and channels, working in harmony to ensure the continuity of our species. Its primary function is to produce, transport, and deliver sperm to the female counterpart for fertilization. But beyond this biological imperative, the system, especially the testicles, has over the ages been emblematic, taking on a broader role in understanding masculinity, cultural norms, and even socio-political dynamics.

The male reproductive system is largely external, setting it apart from its female counterpart. The testes, housed in the scrotum, play the pivotal role of producing the male gametes - sperm - and also the primary male hormone, testosterone. The penile structure is multifunctional; it facilitates the excretion of urine and serves as the conduit for sperm to exit the body during sexual interactions.

Complex as it is, it's not merely the biological function of the male reproductive system that captivates our attention. Its influence spans much further and deeper. Historically, the male reproductive organs, especially the testicles, have been symbolic of power, virility, and vigor. In ancient Rome, for instance, men placed their right hand on their testicles when swearing an oath, leading to the origin of the word "testify". The organ wasn't just a physiological entity, but a beacon of a man's honor, truth, and commitment.

In many African cultures, initiation rites marking the transition from boyhood to manhood often revolved around tests of endurance, resilience, and sometimes even pain, reflecting the societal expectations of male toughness and courage. These rites often used the symbolism of the reproductive system as a cornerstone of male identity.

The cultural significance is also vividly illustrated in art and literature. The Renaissance period, which valued human form in its art, showcased the male anatomy as a symbol of both intellectual and physical strength. Artists like Michelangelo took creative liberty in portraying the male reproductive system, not just as an anatomical study, but as an emblem of divine creation and human potential.

However, the portrayal hasn't always been positive or empowering. In modern times, the male reproductive system has, at times, been subject to mockery, vulnerability, or taboo, reflecting the societal discomfort or unease with discussions around male sexuality or health. This dichotomy between historical reverence and modern discomfort offers a window into the ever-evolving perceptions and cultural complexities surrounding the male reproductive system.

As societies evolve, so does their understanding of what it means to be male. This journey into the 'nuts and bolts' of the male reproductive system is not just an exploration of anatomy and function. It's an endeavor into understanding the very fabric of historical narratives, cultural connotations, and the profound interplay of biology with societal norms. Through this exploration, we embark on a comprehensive quest to demystify and appreciate this crucial aspect of human anatomy, and its broader ramifications in the tapestry of human history and culture.

T he human body is an intricate tapestry of systems and structures, each beautifully designed to fulfill specific roles. Among these, the testicles, a part of the male reproductive system, carry the weight of an entire species' continuity. Nestled within the scrotum, these oval-shaped glands are more than just biological entities; they are reservoirs of life, ensuring the perpetuation of human lineage.

Upon close examination, the testicles reveal themselves to be marvels of anatomical engineering. Their primary function is to produce sperm, the male reproductive cells, and testosterone, the hormone responsible for the development of male secondary sexual characteristics. Each testicle is enveloped in a tough protective layer known as the tunica albuginea, which extends internally to divide the testis into numerous lobules. These lobules house the seminiferous tubules, the site of sperm production, or spermatogenesis. These tubules coil and twist in intricate patterns, and if unraveled, their combined length from just one testicle would measure several meters.

Within these seminiferous tubules, a dance of life takes place. Spermatogonia, the primitive sperm cells, undergo a series of developmental stages, ultimately maturing into the sperm cells that are familiar to us. Alongside this transformative journey, the Sertoli cells, which are also found in the tubules, play the role of nursemaids, nourishing and protecting the developing sperm.

Yet, the journey of the sperm doesn't end in the seminiferous tubules. Once formed, these cells move to the epididymis, a long, coiled tube that sits atop the testicle. It is here that they undergo their final maturation and gain motility. The epididymis serves as a storage chamber, ensuring that the sperm are ready for their eventual journey during ejaculation.

Leading away from the epididymis is the vas deferens, a muscular tube that transports mature sperm to the urethra, from where they are expelled out of the body. Along this pathway, various accessory glands such as the seminal vesicles, prostate gland, and bulbourethral glands contribute seminal fluid. This fluid, combined with sperm, makes up semen, the substance that is ejaculated during sexual climax.

The cooperation between these structures ensures the successful production, maturation, storage, and eventual expulsion of sperm. But beyond this meticulous coordination, these anatomical entities play a role in a man's identity. The testosterone produced in the testicles not only aids in sperm production but is also responsible for the deepening of the voice, the growth of facial and body hair, and the increase in muscle mass during puberty. It shapes the very essence of what society recognizes as 'masculine'.

Understanding the anatomy of the testicles and their associated structures offers more than just a biological perspective. It's a journey into the very heart of life's creation and the complexities that ensure its continuation. The delicate interplay of cells, hormones, and structures within this system is not just a testament to nature's design but also a reflection of the profound miracle that is human reproduction.

L ife, as we know it, begins with the union of two microscopic entities - the egg from the female and the sperm from the male. The latter, albeit smaller in size, embarks on a journey that's nothing short of extraordinary. The story of sperm is one of resilience, precision, and intricate choreography, and understanding this journey takes us deep into the wonders of physiology.

Spermatogenesis, the process through which sperm cells are produced, commences in the testicles, specifically within the coiled labyrinths of the seminiferous tubules. The cycle of sperm production is a marvel of cellular transformation. Starting as spermatogonia, these cells undergo a series of divisions and transformations. First, they replicate their DNA, ensuring that the genetic material is ready to be halved, allowing for the union with the female's egg.

As these cells move closer to the tubular lumen, they differentiate into spermatocytes. Here, a crucial event termed meiosis takes place. Unlike regular cellular divisions, meiosis ensures that the resulting sperm cells have half the typical number of chromosomes. This halving is essential, for when the sperm fuses with the egg, the regular chromosome number is restored, creating a unique blend of both parents' genetic material.

Following meiosis, the spermatocytes further mature into spermatids. At this stage, these cells undergo a dramatic transformation, reshaping and shedding unnecessary components to form a streamlined, motile structure. The result? Mature spermatozoa, with a head containing precious genetic material, a midsection packed with energy-producing mitochondria, and a tail or flagellum that propels them forward.

The newly formed sperm are then ushered into the epididymis, where they mature and acquire the ability to move. This maturation process is essential, for the challenges that lie ahead require strength, endurance, and agility. The sperm's journey, either culminating in fertilization or being expelled from the body, is a testament to nature's intricate design, ensuring that only the fittest reach the destination.

But sperm production is not a solitary act. It's supported and regulated by a symphony of hormones. The hypothalamus in the brain releases gonadotropin-releasing hormone (GnRH). This, in turn, signals the pituitary gland to release two crucial hormones: follicle-stimulating hormone (FSH) and luteinizing hormone (LH). While FSH stimulates the Sertoli cells in the testes, aiding in spermatogenesis, LH acts on the Leydig cells, prompting them to produce testosterone. This hormone not only facilitates sperm production but also plays a pivotal role in maintaining the male's overall reproductive health.

The process of sperm production, guided by a delicate balance of hormones and cellular activities, stands as a testament to the intricacies of human physiology. Each sperm carries with it not just the potential for life but also the legacy of an age-old process, refined over millennia, ensuring the continuation of our species. As we delve deeper into the wonders of the male reproductive system, the profound interplay of structures, cells, and hormones unfolds, painting a picture of nature's unparalleled design.

At the heart of the male reproductive system, beyond the intricate anatomy and delicate processes, lies an even more profound orchestration of hormones. These chemical messengers are the unsung heroes, ensuring that every aspect of male reproduction, from the cellular dances within the testicles to the broader expressions of masculinity, occurs seamlessly. Chief among these hormones, and perhaps the most renowned, is testosterone.

Testosterone, often termed the "male hormone," is responsible for a plethora of functions within the male body. Produced within the interstitial cells, or Leydig cells, of the testicles, its influence is felt far beyond the boundaries of the reproductive system. From the onset of puberty, testosterone shapes the male physique, deepening the voice, stimulating the growth of facial and body hair, enhancing muscle mass, and influencing fat distribution. But its role doesn't stop at physical attributes. It plays a pivotal role in influencing male behavior, modulating moods, and even impacting cognitive functions.

However, testosterone production and regulation is a finely tuned process. The hypothalamus and pituitary gland, both nestled within the brain, serve as the maestros of this hormonal symphony. The hypothalamus, sensing the levels of circulating testosterone, releases the gonadotropin-releasing hormone (GnRH). This prompts the pituitary gland to secrete luteinizing hormone (LH) and, to a lesser extent, follicle-stimulating hormone (FSH). While LH stimulates the production of testosterone in the Leydig cells, FSH, in tandem with testosterone, supports spermatogenesis.

But testosterone doesn't work in isolation. A host of other hormones play supportive roles. For instance, dihydrotestosterone (DHT), a derivative of testosterone, is vital for the development of primary and secondary male sexual characteristics. Another hormone, inhibin, released by the Sertoli cells in the testes, acts as a regulator, providing feedback to the pituitary gland about sperm production rates and influencing the release of FSH.

This hormonal dance is not static. It changes with the rhythms of life. Testosterone levels, for instance, naturally peak during adolescence and early adulthood and gradually decline as men age. This decline, often referred to as 'andropause', is accompanied by a range of physiological changes, akin to the more widely discussed female menopause.

The equilibrium of the hormonal milieu is delicate. Disruptions, be it due to medical conditions, external factors, or lifestyle choices, can have profound effects on the male reproductive system and overall health. Conditions such as hypogonadism, where the body doesn't produce enough testosterone, can affect everything from bone density to mood and libido.

In essence, while the structures of the male reproductive system are the tangible entities we often focus on, the hormones are the invisible threads weaving the tapestry of male physiology and identity. As we journey through the complexities of the male reproductive system, it becomes evident that understanding the hormonal milieu is not just about appreciating the chemicals at play, but about recognizing the profound ways in which they shape the essence of male existence.

The marvel that is the male reproductive system, with its intricate anatomy and harmonious hormonal play, is not without its susceptibilities. Just as every complex system can face disruptions, the testicles, despite their protective housing within the scrotum, are prone to various disorders and diseases. An exploration of these vulnerabilities not only paints a holistic picture of male reproductive health but also emphasizes the importance of awareness and timely medical interventions.

One of the most common issues faced by men of varying ages is testicular torsion. This acute and painful condition occurs when the spermatic cord, which provides blood flow to the testicle, twists and cuts off the blood supply. Immediate medical attention is essential, for a prolonged lack of blood can lead to permanent damage to the testicle.

In tandem with torsion, epididymitis, or inflammation of the epididymis, presents itself as a frequent ailment. Often caused by bacterial infections, it results in pain and swelling and can be addressed with antibiotics. If left untreated, however, it might lead to complications, including abscess formation and even infertility.

But perhaps the most discussed and feared disease associated with the testicles is testicular cancer. While relatively rare compared to other cancers, its incidence in younger men makes it a significant concern. Manifesting often as a painless lump or swelling in the testicles, early detection is crucial. With advancements in medical science, the prognosis for testicular cancer has significantly improved, and many men go on to live full, healthy lives post-treatment.

While the above conditions are among the more commonly known, several other disorders can affect the testicles. Varicoceles, for instance, are enlarged veins in the scrotum, akin to varicose veins one might see in the legs. They can cause pain, swelling, and even have implications for fertility. Similarly, hydroceles and spermatoceles, fluid-filled sacs around the testicle, might require medical attention if they grow large or become painful.

Beyond these physical ailments, hormonal imbalances, such as reduced testosterone levels, can affect the testicles' function and have broader implications for a man's health and well-being. Symptoms can range from fatigue and reduced libido to more severe manifestations like osteoporosis.

In the realm of male reproductive health, awareness is paramount. Regular self-examinations, much like breast examinations in women, can be invaluable in early detection of testicular issues. Recognizing changes, be it in size, shape, or the onset of pain, and seeking medical advice, can be life-saving.

While the vulnerabilities of the testicles might seem daunting, they offer a perspective on the delicate balance of the male reproductive system. As with all aspects of health, understanding potential risks underscores the significance of prevention, regular check-ups, and timely interventions. In the grand tapestry of the male reproductive system, acknowledging vulnerabilities is as essential as celebrating its marvels, for it fosters a comprehensive appreciation of the male physiological journey.

L ife's most profound miracle is perhaps the creation of a new being, a process that hinges on the collaboration between the male and female reproductive systems. Central to this interplay is the role of the testicles in ensuring fertility. A journey into the realm of male fertility is not just about understanding the mechanics of sperm production but also about appreciating the intricate factors that influence the viability and health of these microscopic entities.

Every sperm carries with it the promise of life, but for successful fertilization to occur, several criteria must be met. Firstly, there's the matter of quantity. A typical ejaculation releases tens of millions of sperm, and yet, only a fraction will even approach the egg, with only one achieving the honor of fertilization. This vast number ensures a fighting chance against the many hurdles that await in the female reproductive tract.

But quantity without quality is futile. The health of the sperm, from its genetic material to its motility - the ability to move efficiently towards the egg - is paramount. Morphology, or the shape and structure of the sperm, also plays a significant role. Misshapen sperm, or those with structural anomalies, might find the journey to the egg challenging, if not impossible.

The testicles ensure both the production and health of sperm, but several external factors can influence their efficacy. Environmental toxins, excessive heat, certain medications, and even lifestyle choices like smoking and excessive alcohol consumption can adversely affect sperm health. In some cases, genetic factors or underlying medical conditions might be at play, affecting both the quantity and quality of sperm produced.

A decrease in fertility potential, often termed male infertility, can be multifaceted. While sperm health is a significant factor, issues like blockages in the vas deferens, which prevent the release of sperm, or hormonal imbalances that affect sperm production can also contribute. Understanding the root of the problem is crucial, for it paves the way for targeted interventions, from lifestyle changes to medical procedures.

In the modern era, with increasing awareness and technological advancements, addressing male fertility has become more nuanced. Medical science now offers a plethora of diagnostic tools, from semen analysis to genetic screenings, to pinpoint issues. Furthermore, treatments ranging from medications and surgeries to assisted reproductive technologies like in vitro fertilization (IVF) provide hope to countless couples aspiring for parenthood.

Yet, the conversation around fertility transcends the biological. Societal perceptions, emotional implications, and the weight of legacy and lineage often interweave with the clinical. For many men, fertility challenges can lead to feelings of inadequacy or a perceived loss of masculinity. Thus, addressing male fertility is not just about medical interventions but also about holistic support, encompassing emotional and psychological well-being.

In the grand narrative of the male reproductive system, the testicles' role in procreation stands as a testament to nature's desire for continuity. As we journey through the myriad facets of male reproductive health, recognizing the profound interplay of biology, environment, and emotion in the realm of fertility offers a deeper understanding of the challenges, triumphs, and miracles that color the human reproductive saga.

T ime, in its inexorable march, leaves no aspect of human physiology untouched, and the male reproductive system is no exception. As men age, the testicles, like other organs, undergo a series of transformations, reflecting the broader changes in the body. Delving into the nuances of these shifts provides not only a biological perspective but also a profound insight into the ebb and flow of life itself.

The journey begins in adolescence. Puberty heralds the awakening of the testicles, with a surge in testosterone production driving the development of secondary sexual characteristics. This period sees the testicles grow in size, marking the onset of sperm production and the capability for reproduction. It's a phase of rapid change, mirrored by the emotional and psychological transitions typical of teenage years.

However, as the exuberance of youth gives way to the steadiness of adulthood, the testicles settle into a more consistent rhythm. Testosterone levels stabilize, ensuring the maintenance of male characteristics and supporting overall health. Fertility reaches its peak, with the quality and quantity of sperm production being optimal.

But as with all things in nature, this equilibrium is not perpetual. Beginning in the late 30s and more markedly in the 40s and beyond, men experience a gradual decline in testosterone levels. Termed the "andropause" or "male menopause," this phase mirrors the more dramatic hormonal shifts seen in women during menopause. The effects, though subtler, are palpable. There's a reduction in muscle mass and bone density, a subtle shift in fat distribution, and potential changes in mood and libido. Energy levels might wane, and cognitive functions could show signs of slowing.

Concurrently, sperm quality starts to exhibit changes. While men continue to produce sperm well into old age, the genetic integrity of these cells can be compromised. Research indicates that children of older fathers face a slightly increased risk of certain health conditions, emphasizing the importance of genetic health in the context of reproduction.

Beyond hormonal and reproductive changes, the testicles become more vulnerable to certain ailments with age. The risk of testicular cancer, though still low, can increase. Prostate health, closely linked to the testicular function, also becomes a focus, with prostate enlargement or benign prostatic hyperplasia (BPH) affecting many men in their 60s and beyond.

Yet, while the biological narrative of aging paints a picture of decline, it's essential to view it in the broader context of life's journey. Aging brings with it wisdom, experience, and often, a sense of contentment and perspective. Modern medicine, coupled with a greater understanding of health and well-being, ensures that many of the challenges of aging can be managed, if not mitigated.

In the continuum of the male reproductive system's story, the chapter on aging stands as a poignant reminder of life's impermanence and beauty. As we traverse the myriad phases of male reproductive health, understanding the nuances of aging offers a holistic view, interweaving biology, emotion, and the profound mysteries of existence.

In the intricate tapestry of life, every thread is interconnected. The male reproductive system, with its multifaceted structures and functions, is not an isolated entity. Instead, it is profoundly influenced by the broader lifestyle choices and environmental exposures that color every individual's journey. Unraveling these connections illuminates not only the vulnerabilities of the testicles but also the proactive measures men can adopt to ensure optimal health.

Diet, often touted as the cornerstone of well-being, has significant implications for testicular health. The nutrients consumed directly impact the production of hormones and sperm quality. For instance, diets rich in antioxidants, such as Vitamin C and E, have been associated with improved sperm health, safeguarding these cells from oxidative stress. Conversely, excessive consumption of processed foods and those high in saturated fats can negatively impact testosterone levels and overall reproductive function.

Physical activity, another pillar of holistic health, plays a dual role. Regular exercise can boost testosterone production, enhancing libido and overall energy levels. However, specific activities, like prolonged cycling, have been noted to potentially impact sperm quality due to the increased testicular temperature and pressure. Balance, as with many aspects of life, is the key.

The modern world, with its myriad conveniences, also brings along a suite of challenges. Stress, an almost ubiquitous aspect of contemporary living, can have detrimental effects on the testicles. Chronic stress leads to elevated cortisol levels, which can suppress testosterone production. Over time, this can lead to diminished libido, reduced sperm quality, and broader health issues.

No discussion of lifestyle would be complete without addressing the impact of substances like alcohol, tobacco, and recreational drugs. Excessive alcohol consumption can reduce testosterone levels, impairing sperm production. Smoking, with its myriad toxins, has been linked to reduced sperm count and compromised sperm health. Recreational drugs, depending on their nature, can disrupt hormonal balance and affect reproductive function.

Environmental factors, too, play a role. Exposure to certain toxins, like heavy metals and pesticides, can diminish sperm health. Similarly, prolonged exposure to heat, such as in saunas or through occupations like welding, can temporarily reduce sperm count.

However, the narrative isn't solely about vulnerabilities. It's also about empowerment. Awareness of these influences allows men to make informed choices, be it in diet, activity, or stress management. Moreover, with the advancements in medical science, many of the effects of lifestyle choices on testicular health can be mitigated or reversed.

In the broader story of the male reproductive system, the chapter on lifestyle stands as a testament to the interconnectedness of life. It emphasizes that the choices made every day, from the food consumed to the way stress is managed, ripple through the body, impacting every organ, including the testicles. As we navigate the complexities of male reproductive health, recognizing these interconnections offers a roadmap for proactive care and holistic well-being.

The human body, in its vast complexity, is governed by a series of messengers, with hormones taking center stage. Among these, testosterone, predominantly produced in the testicles, stands as a symbol of masculinity, influencing a myriad of physiological processes beyond just the male reproductive system. Delving deep into the world of testosterone offers a glimpse into its multifaceted role, its interplay with other hormones, and its significance in the broader tapestry of male health.

Often dubbed the 'male hormone,' testosterone drives the development of male secondary sexual characteristics. From the deepening of the voice during puberty, the growth of facial and body hair, to the development of muscle mass, its influence is palpable. But beyond these visible manifestations, testosterone plays a subtler, yet equally crucial role in maintaining bone density, red blood cell production, and the overall sense of well-being in men.

Yet, testosterone does not act in isolation. Its production and release are orchestrated by a harmonious interplay of hormones, beginning in the brain. The hypothalamus releases gonadotropin-releasing hormone (GnRH), which signals the pituitary gland to produce luteinizing hormone (LH) and follicle-stimulating hormone (FSH). While LH prompts the testicles to produce testosterone, FSH collaborates with testosterone to facilitate sperm production. This elegant dance ensures a balanced and coordinated reproductive function.

However, like all physiological processes, this hormonal dance can face disruptions. Low testosterone levels, or hypogonadism, can arise from various causes. Primary hypogonadism pertains to issues with the testicles themselves, which might be due to genetic factors, injury, or other conditions like mumps orchitis. In contrast, secondary hypogonadism arises from problems in the hypothalamus or pituitary gland, affecting the release of GnRH or LH and FSH, respectively.

The ramifications of low testosterone levels can be broad and varied. Physically, men might experience reduced muscle mass, increased body fat, and diminished bone density. The effects, however, aren't limited to the tangible. Reduced libido, fatigue, mood disturbances, and even cognitive changes can manifest, emphasizing the profound influence of testosterone on overall health.

Modern medicine offers a plethora of diagnostic tools to assess testosterone levels and pinpoint underlying causes. Blood tests provide a quantitative measure, while imaging tests and genetic screenings can provide insights into potential root causes. Furthermore, treatments like testosterone replacement therapy (TRT) have offered hope and improved quality of life for many men with hypogonadism. However, as with all interventions, a nuanced understanding of the benefits and potential risks is crucial.

The narrative of testosterone, in the grand journey of the male reproductive system, underscores the profound interconnectedness of the body's processes. Recognizing its multifaceted role, the delicate balance it maintains with other hormones, and its broader implications on health, offers a holistic understanding of male physiology. As we explore the depths of male reproductive health, appreciating the dance of hormones enriches the perspective, emphasizing the harmony and balance that define the human experience.

eep within the folds of the male reproductive system lie potential vulnerabilities, manifestations of which can ripple through an individual's physical and emotional life. These silent struggles, encompassing a range of testicular health disorders, shed light on the delicate balance that sustains reproductive and overall well-being. Unearthing these conditions, their causes, and implications provides a comprehensive insight into the challenges some men face, emphasizing the importance of awareness, early detection, and effective management.

Testicular torsion stands as one of the most acute emergencies in male reproductive health. It involves the twisting of the spermatic cord, cutting off blood supply to the testicle. Swift intervention is paramount, for a delay can lead to permanent damage or loss of the affected testicle. The onset is typically sudden, characterized by severe pain and swelling. While the exact cause remains elusive, certain anatomical factors may predispose an individual to torsion.

Varicocele, on the other hand, is a more chronic condition, likened to varicose veins but located within the scrotum. These enlarged veins can disrupt the temperature regulation of the testicles, potentially impairing sperm production and quality. Men might remain asymptomatic, or experience discomfort and swelling. While not life-threatening, varicoceles can impact fertility and warrant monitoring or intervention.

Hydrocele and spermatocele are conditions related to fluid accumulation. The former involves fluid buildup around the testicle, leading to scrotal swelling, while the latter pertains to a cyst in the epididymis filled with fluid and sperm. Both conditions are typically painless, with treatment considerations based on size, discomfort, or associated complications.

Testicular cancer, although relatively rare, holds significance due to its potential impact on young men. Often presenting as a painless lump in the testicle, it requires prompt diagnosis and intervention. The prognosis for testicular cancer remains promising, especially when detected early, with treatments ranging from surgery to chemotherapy and radiation.

Beyond the physical manifestations, it's crucial to recognize the emotional and psychological toll of these conditions. Fertility concerns, body image issues, and the weight of a potential diagnosis can exert immense stress on an individual. The importance of holistic care, encompassing not just medical interventions but also emotional support, cannot be overstated.

In the expansive narrative of the male reproductive system, the chapter on testicular health disorders emphasizes the vulnerabilities that lie beneath the surface. Yet, with increased awareness, proactive healthcare measures, and advancements in medical science, many of these challenges can be surmounted. As we continue our exploration of male reproductive health, understanding these silent struggles underscores the resilience of the human spirit, the importance of support, and the undying hope that defines the human experience.

In the intricate symphony of life, reproduction stands as one of its most profound expressions. Yet, for many, this dance is fraught with challenges, with male infertility emerging as a poignant theme. While traditionally women bore the weight of fertility concerns, the modern understanding emphasizes that fertility is a shared journey. Diving deep into the nuances of male infertility offers a comprehensive view of its causes, implications, and the road to potential solutions.

At its core, male infertility pertains to the inability to cause a pregnancy, despite consistent and unprotected intercourse. It's a multifaceted issue, with causes spanning anatomical, hormonal, genetic, and environmental factors.

Sperm quality and quantity lie at the heart of reproductive capability. Azoospermia, or the complete absence of sperm in the semen, presents a clear challenge. This condition can arise from obstructive causes, such as blockages in the ductal system, or non-obstructive ones like impaired sperm production. On the other hand, oligospermia refers to reduced sperm concentration, which can be influenced by factors ranging from hormonal imbalances to varicoceles.

Beyond sheer numbers, the functionality and structure of sperm are paramount.

Motility, or the ability of sperm to move efficiently, is crucial for reaching and penetrating the egg. Teratospermia, a condition characterized by a high percentage of abnormally shaped sperm, can impede the fertilization process. Both these factors, often assessed through a semen analysis, play pivotal roles in determining fertility potential.

Hormonal imbalances, as discussed in previous chapters, can directly impact sperm production and overall reproductive health. Reduced testosterone levels or imbalances in FSH and LH can compromise the testicles' ability to produce healthy sperm. Moreover, genetic disorders like Klinefelter syndrome can disrupt normal testicular development and function.

Environmental and lifestyle factors, too, interweave into the narrative of male infertility. Chronic exposure to certain toxins, excessive alcohol consumption, smoking, and even certain medications can impair sperm health. The role of stress, with its potential to disrupt hormonal balance, cannot be understated.

However, amidst the challenges, there's a beacon of hope. Modern reproductive medicine has made leaps and bounds in diagnosing and managing male infertility. Techniques ranging from sperm retrieval procedures for those with azoospermia to advanced assisted reproductive technologies like intracytoplasmic sperm injection (ICSI) offer a glimmer of hope to many couples.

Beyond the medical dimension, the emotional landscape of infertility is profound. Feelings of inadequacy, guilt, and frustration can cloud the journey, highlighting the need for comprehensive care. Support groups, counseling, and open communication between partners become invaluable pillars during this journey.

In the grand chronicle of the male reproductive system, the chapter on male infertility stands as a testament to the complexities of reproduction. Recognizing its multi-faceted nature, the advances in medical science, and the emotional depth of the experience offers a holistic view of this silent struggle. As we further traverse the vast terrain of male reproductive health, understanding infertility underscores the delicate balance of life and the unwavering human spirit that seeks to nurture it.

In the intricate journey of understanding the male reproductive system, one principle resonates with unwavering clarity: prevention is paramount. Just as a skilled gardener nurtures every plant with attention and care, ensuring optimal health for the male reproductive system necessitates proactive measures and cultivated habits. Delving into these practices offers a guide for fostering health, preventing potential disorders, and ensuring the vitality of the system that plays such a pivotal role in human life.

Diet emerges as one of the cornerstones of testicular and reproductive health. A well-balanced diet, rich in antioxidants, minerals, and essential fatty acids, can enhance sperm quality and bolster overall reproductive health. Foods rich in zinc, selenium, and Vitamin E, such as nuts, seeds, and green leafy vegetables, are particularly beneficial. Omega-3 fatty acids, found abundantly in fish like salmon, play a role in improving sperm membrane fluidity, facilitating their function.

Hydration, often overlooked, is another vital aspect. Adequate water intake ensures the right consistency of semen and supports the proper functioning of cells within the testicles. Reducing excessive caffeine and alcohol consumption is also advisable, as both can impact sperm quality when consumed in large quantities.

Physical activity and its influence on the male reproductive system present a nuanced narrative. Regular exercise can enhance testosterone production and improve overall health, which indirectly benefits reproductive function. However, moderation is key. Overexertion can elevate cortisol levels, potentially suppressing testosterone. Furthermore, wearing protective gear during contact sports is essential to prevent testicular injuries.

Temperature regulation, particularly for the testicles, is of paramount importance. Prolonged exposure to elevated temperatures, whether from tight clothing, frequent sauna visits, or occupations involving high heat, can temporarily impact sperm production. Thus, making conscious choices, like wearing loose-fitting underwear and taking breaks from constant heat exposure, can be beneficial.

Regular medical check-ups, including testicular self-exams, play a proactive role in early detection of potential issues. Early diagnosis, be it for conditions like testicular cancer or infections, often results in more effective treatments and better outcomes.

Stress management, given its profound influence on hormonal balance and overall well-being, emerges as an essential aspect of nurturing reproductive health. Engaging in relaxation techniques like meditation, deep breathing exercises, or even hobbies can significantly mitigate the impact of chronic stress.

Avoiding harmful substances, from recreational drugs to certain medications without medical supervision, further contributes to the health of the male reproductive system. Being aware of potential toxins in the environment, like pesticides or heavy metals, and minimizing exposure can also safeguard against their detrimental effects.

In the vast narrative of the male reproductive system, the chapter on preventative measures and healthy habits underscores the adage that an ounce of prevention is worth a pound of cure. Recognizing the profound influence of daily choices, from the food consumed to the methods of stress management, provides a roadmap for a healthy and fulfilling reproductive journey. As we continue to navigate the complexities of male reproductive health, embracing these nurturing practices illuminates the path toward vitality, longevity, and well-being.

In the vast tapestry of human history, the understanding and valuation of male fertility have ebbed and flowed, carving unique impressions across cultures, societies, and epochs. Unraveling these historical perspectives reveals a rich mosaic of beliefs, practices, and traditions, offering a deeper appreciation of the intricate relationship between man and his reproductive capacity.

Ancient civilizations, teeming with myths and legends, wove the essence of fertility into their very fabric. In Ancient Egypt, the god Min, often depicted with an erect phallus, symbolized fertility and male sexual prowess. Festivals honoring Min, replete with singing, dancing, and merriment, showcased the reverence for male reproductive potency in this era.

In stark contrast, the Greco-Roman world approached male fertility with a blend of scientific curiosity and moral philosophy. The famed physician Hippocrates posited that both men and women contributed 'seeds' to the creation of offspring, challenging earlier notions that solely credited women for the character and traits of the progeny. Meanwhile, Roman society often linked virility with virtues of strength, courage, and honor, creating an interplay between reproductive capacity and moral character.

Asia's rich tapestry of cultures brought its own color to the spectrum. Ancient Chinese texts, notably the Yellow Emperor's Classic of Internal Medicine, elaborated on the concept of 'jing' or essence, which represented the life force and was closely tied to male reproductive vitality. Preserving and nurturing this 'jing' through practices like acupuncture, herbal remedies, and meditation became central to traditional Chinese medicine.

India's ancient Ayurvedic system approached male fertility with a holistic lens. The concept of 'Shukra dhatu' or seminal tissue was integral to reproductive health. Imbalances or deficiencies in this tissue, it was believed, could be addressed through specific dietary practices, herbs, and even yogic exercises. The famous Kama Sutra, while primarily a guide to love and pleasure, also touched upon aspects of fertility and procreation.

The Middle Ages in Europe brought a shift in understanding and attitude. With the Church's rise in influence, topics related to reproduction and sexuality often met with caution, if not outright repression. However, this period also saw the advent of early medical treatises that began exploring male reproductive disorders, albeit with a blend of fact and superstition.

The Renaissance, true to its spirit of rebirth, rejuvenated interest in human anatomy and physiology. Pioneers like Andreas Vesalius began documenting the male reproductive system with unprecedented detail, laying the groundwork for modern urology and andrology.

As the pages of history turned to the modern era, the intersection of science and technology propelled our understanding of male fertility to new heights. The invention of the microscope revealed the enigmatic world of sperm, and scientific breakthroughs shed light on the complexities of male reproductive health.

In this journey through time, the perceptions and practices surrounding male fertility showcase the evolution of human thought, belief, and understanding. As we stand on the shoulders of giants, gazing into the horizons of the future, these whispers of the past remind us of the enduring bond between mankind and the mysteries of reproduction. As we forge ahead, charting the frontiers of male reproductive health, these historical insights anchor us, infusing our quest with depth, context, and reverence.

The vast expanse of the male reproductive system, while deeply rooted in the tangible realm of biology, is intimately interwoven with the intricate tapestries of the mind. It's a dance between the physiological and the psychological, where the ebbs and flows of emotions, perceptions, and beliefs play a pivotal role in shaping reproductive well-being.

For eons, emotions like stress, anxiety, and depression have cast their shadows on the realm of male fertility. Stress, often dubbed the silent killer of modern times, has a profound influence on the reproductive system. Chronic stress leads to the sustained release of cortisol, a hormone that can interfere with the production of testosterone. This delicate balance between stress hormones and reproductive hormones underscores the inextricable link between the mind's turmoil and physiological function.

Anxiety, too, weaves its tendrils into the fabric of reproductive health. Performance anxiety, often stemming from societal pressures and self-imposed standards, can lead to erectile issues. The cyclical nature of anxiety ensures that one such episode often fuels apprehensions about future encounters, creating a self-perpetuating cycle that can be debilitating.

Depression, with its heavy cloak of despair, impacts reproductive health in myriad ways. Reduced libido, one of the hallmarks of depressive disorders, directly affects reproductive potential. Furthermore, many antidepressant medications can have side effects that impact erectile function or semen quality, adding another layer to this intricate puzzle.

But the psychological domain's influence isn't confined merely to these broad-brush emotions. Self-perception and self-worth play crucial roles in shaping reproductive health. Societal constructs often link virility with masculinity, and challenges like infertility or reproductive disorders can lead to feelings of inadequacy or diminished self-worth. Such emotional turbulence, if unchecked, can further exacerbate reproductive challenges.

Cultural and familial expectations, particularly in societies where progeny is given paramount importance, can also impact male reproductive health. The perceived 'duty' to continue family lines or to meet societal benchmarks can place immense psychological pressure on individuals, creating a milieu ripe for reproductive challenges.

Yet, amidst the challenges, the mind's resilience and adaptability shine through. Psychotherapy and counseling emerge as potent tools to navigate the stormy seas of reproductive challenges. Cognitive-behavioral therapy, in particular, offers strategies to reshape negative thought patterns and foster a more positive and proactive outlook. Support groups, by creating a space for shared experiences and mutual understanding, offer solace and camaraderie.

Mindfulness practices, like meditation and deep breathing, offer an oasis of calm, helping regulate stress and nurture a balanced mental space. In tandem with medical interventions, these practices ensure a comprehensive approach to reproductive health, considering both the body's intricacies and the mind's profundities.

In the ongoing narrative of male reproductive health, recognizing the mind-body confluence offers a holistic and nuanced perspective. It's a reminder that the journey isn't merely physiological but is deeply intertwined with the emotions, beliefs, and perceptions that shape human existence. As we venture deeper into the labyrinth of the male reproductive system, acknowledging this intricate dance between mind and body enriches our understanding, fostering a more compassionate, informed, and holistic approach to well-being.

N estled within the vast symphony of the human body, hormones play the subtle notes that orchestrate a range of functions, from growth and metabolism to mood and reproduction. Often overlooked in their quiet elegance, these chemical messengers wield formidable influence, ensuring the harmonious interplay of various bodily systems. In the realm of male reproduction, understanding these silent rhythms is pivotal, for they are the unseen conductors guiding the dance of fertility and vitality.

At the heart of male reproductive health stands testosterone, the primary male sex hormone. Produced predominantly in the testicles, testosterone serves myriad roles, from driving the development of male reproductive tissues during fetal life to fostering the secondary sexual characteristics that emerge during puberty. This includes the deepening of the voice, the sprouting of facial and body hair, and the growth of the Adam's apple. As men transition from adolescence to adulthood, testosterone continues its guardianship, maintaining sperm production, libido, and overall virility.

Yet, the hormonal tapestry is richer than just testosterone. Luteinizing hormone (LH) and follicle-stimulating hormone (FSH), produced in the anterior pituitary gland, are central players in the symphony of male reproduction. While LH spurs the testicles to produce testosterone, FSH collaborates with testosterone to facilitate the production of sperm. These hormones, in their intricate dance, ensure that the testicles function optimally, producing both viable sperm and adequate testosterone.

Prolactin, another hormone stemming from the pituitary gland, albeit lesser-known, has an influential role in male reproductive health. Elevated levels can adversely impact testosterone production and potentially lead to reproductive challenges. Factors like certain medications, pituitary tumors, or even prolonged stress can result in elevated prolactin, underscoring the delicate balance of the hormonal milieu.

Thyroid hormones, primarily known for their role in metabolism, have a subtle but significant influence on male reproductive health. Imbalances, either an underactive or overactive thyroid, can impact testosterone levels, sperm quality, and even libido. It is a testament to the intricate interplay of various hormonal systems, each influencing the other in ways both profound and nuanced.

Adrenal hormones, particularly cortisol, often dubbed the 'stress hormone', also leave their mark on the landscape of male reproduction. Chronic stress, leading to sustained elevated cortisol levels, can suppress testosterone production, creating a ripple effect that impacts various facets of male reproductive health.

In navigating the labyrinth of male reproductive health, understanding these silent rhythms is pivotal. Hormonal imbalances, be they subtle or pronounced, can give rise to a range of challenges, from infertility and reduced libido to broader issues like fatigue or mood disturbances. Thus, regular screenings, particularly as one ages or experiences reproductive challenges, become essential.

Modern medicine, with its advancements, offers a range of interventions to address hormonal imbalances. From hormone replacement therapies and medications to lifestyle interventions, the toolkit is vast and varied. Yet, the first step always remains understanding – recognizing the silent symphony, the delicate dance of hormones that shapes the panorama of male reproductive health.

In this chapter, as we have delved into the world of hormones, it's evident that the dance of reproduction is both intricate and profound. These silent rhythms, though often overlooked, form the very foundation of vitality, fertility, and well-being. As we continue to unravel the mysteries of the male reproductive system, this hormonal tapestry serves as a gentle reminder of the delicate balances and profound interconnections that define human existence.

The journey of male reproduction, while deeply influenced by the inner workings of physiology and psychology, is also swayed by external forces. The environment we inhabit, the choices we make, the lifestyles we adopt

– all leave indelible marks on the intricate canvas of reproductive health. Exploring these influences offers a holistic perspective, emphasizing the delicate balance between the inner self and the external world.

Air, water, and soil, the triad that sustains life, bear witness to the footprints of modern civilization. Industrialization, while propelling humanity to unprecedented heights, has also left its residues in the form of pollutants. Chemicals like phthalates, bisphenol A (BPA), and heavy metals, often found in plastics, cosmetics, and even certain foods, have been linked to reduced sperm quality and altered testosterone levels. Their insidious presence in daily life makes them particularly challenging to avoid, highlighting the need for awareness and proactive measures.

Electromagnetic radiation, a relatively recent concern, has garnered attention for its potential impact on male reproductive health. Devices we've grown reliant upon, like mobile phones and laptops, emit low levels of radiation.

While research is still in its nascent stages, prolonged exposure, especially when devices are kept close to the reproductive organs, has raised concerns about sperm quality and viability.

The food we consume and the beverages we sip play a pivotal role in shaping reproductive health. Diets rich in processed foods, laden with sugars and unhealthy fats, can impact testosterone levels and overall sperm health. Conversely, diets abundant in antioxidants, omega-3 fatty acids, and micronutrients can bolster sperm quality and improve hormonal balance. Alcohol, when consumed in excess, can impact testosterone production, while smoking has been linked to reduced sperm count and motility.

Physical activity, that timeless elixir of health, plays a dual role in male reproductive well-being. Regular exercise can enhance testosterone levels, improve mood, and optimize overall health, all beneficial for reproductive prowess. Yet, excesses, like overly intense training without adequate recovery, can temporarily depress testosterone levels, emphasizing the need for balance.

Emotional well-being, deeply intertwined with lifestyle choices, also casts its influence. Chronic stress, sleep deprivation, and unresolved emotional traumas can create hormonal imbalances, reduce libido, and even impact sperm health. Finding outlets for relaxation, whether through hobbies, meditation, or deep connections, becomes not just a pursuit of mental peace but also of reproductive well-being.

Substance use, particularly anabolic steroids for muscle building or recreational drugs, can have profound effects on the reproductive system. Steroids, by introducing external testosterone, can suppress the body's natural production, leading to testicular shrinkage and reduced sperm production. Recreational drugs, depending on their nature and extent of use, can have varied impacts, from hormonal imbalances to direct effects on sperm health.

In charting the vast seascape of male reproductive health, it becomes evident that the external world, with its myriad influences, plays a role as pivotal as the internal symphony of hormones, emotions, and cellular mechanisms. Recognizing these influences, making informed choices, and seeking balance become the guiding stars, illuminating the path to optimal reproductive well-being.

In this exploration, it's evident that while nature has its designs and rhythms, the choices and environments that modern life presents shape, challenge, and sometimes redefine these natural cadences. Navigating this delicate balance requires awareness, informed choices, and sometimes, a return to the basics – clean air, pure water, nourishing food, and emotional harmony. As we continue our journey through the intricacies of the male reproductive system, this chapter serves as a reminder of the profound interplay between man, his choices, and the world he inhabits.

Every journey, while distinct in its waypoints and landscapes, culminates in a moment of reflection, a pause to appreciate the intricate tapestry woven from experiences, discoveries, and emotions.

Our voyage through the world of male reproductive health, expansive and profound, beckons such a moment, an opportunity to behold the beauty and complexity of this quintessential aspect of human existence.

At its very core, the male reproductive system, with its myriad structures and functions, is a testament to the wonders of biology. The intricate dance of hormones, the silent rhythms of cellular processes, the delicate balance of emotions and physiology – all converge to create a system that, in its essence, transcends the individual. It speaks to the legacy of generations, the promise of progeny, and the eternal cycle of life.

Our exploration has underscored the profound interplay of internal and external forces. The mind's depths, with its reservoirs of emotions, beliefs, and perceptions, influence the reproductive dance as much as the tangible world of anatomy and physiology. Similarly, the choices we make, the environments we inhabit, and the lifestyles we adopt cast their shadows and shine their lights on this intricate canvas.

Yet, beyond the realms of science, beyond the corridors of medicine and research, lies a narrative that's deeply personal and profoundly universal. The journey of male reproduction is not just about the mechanics of procreation. It's about identity and masculinity, about legacy and lineage, about the age-old desires to connect, to belong, and to continue. It's a narrative interwoven with love and longing, hope and despair, joy and sorrow.

In this modern age, where science and technology offer insights and interventions like never before, it's essential to remember the sanctity of the individual journey. Every challenge faced, every joy experienced, every hope harbored in the realm of reproductive health is unique. While collective wisdom guides, individual narratives define.

As we conclude this exploration, it's also a moment to look ahead, to envision a world where understanding is deeper, compassion is greater, and care is more holistic. Where societal constructs and pressures don't define virility or worth. Where every individual, irrespective of their reproductive capacities or challenges, is celebrated for their essence, their spirit, their humanity.

In the end, the tapestry of male reproductive health is but a fragment of the grand mosaic of human existence. Yet, it's a fragment that captures the essence of life itself – the rhythms of creation, the cycles of time, and the eternal dance of legacy.

And so, with gratitude for the knowledge garnered and hope for the journeys ahead, we close this chapter, not as an end, but as a beginning. A beginning of deeper understanding, greater compassion, and a more harmonious dance with the rhythms of life.